ME and JUBILEE

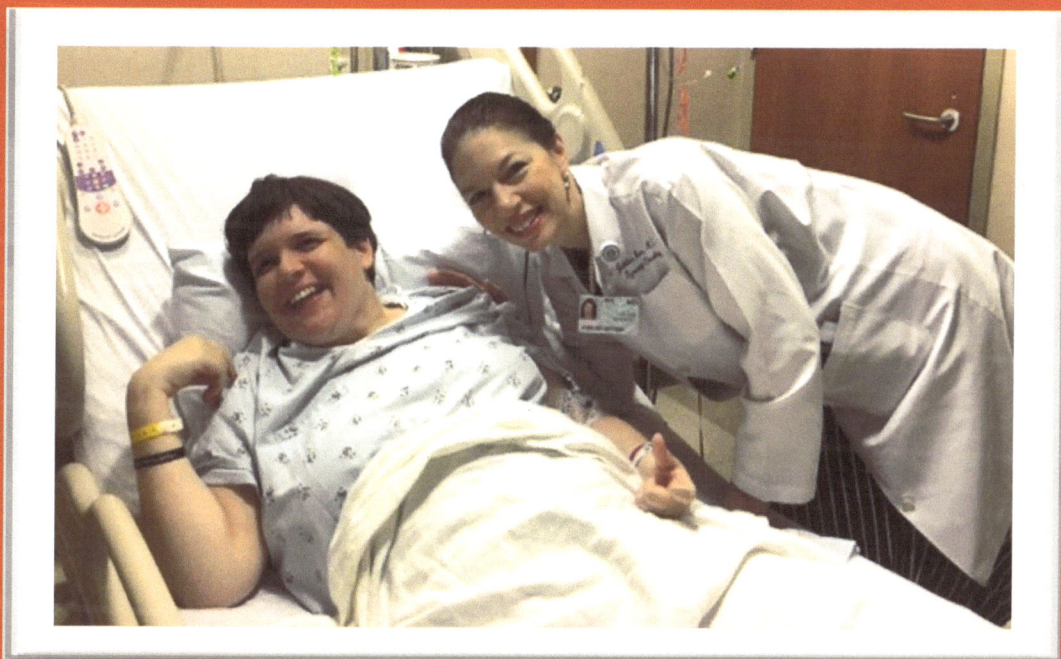

JERYL CHRISTMAS

This Book Belongs To

_____

Thanks to the doctors and nurses at
CMC Pineville, CMC Main,
Levine Cancer Institute, MedCenter Air,
and a very special thanks to
Dr. Jubilee Brown.

Are you nervous seeing doctors,
or sometimes are you scared?
Then let me tell you of MY time
to help you be prepared …

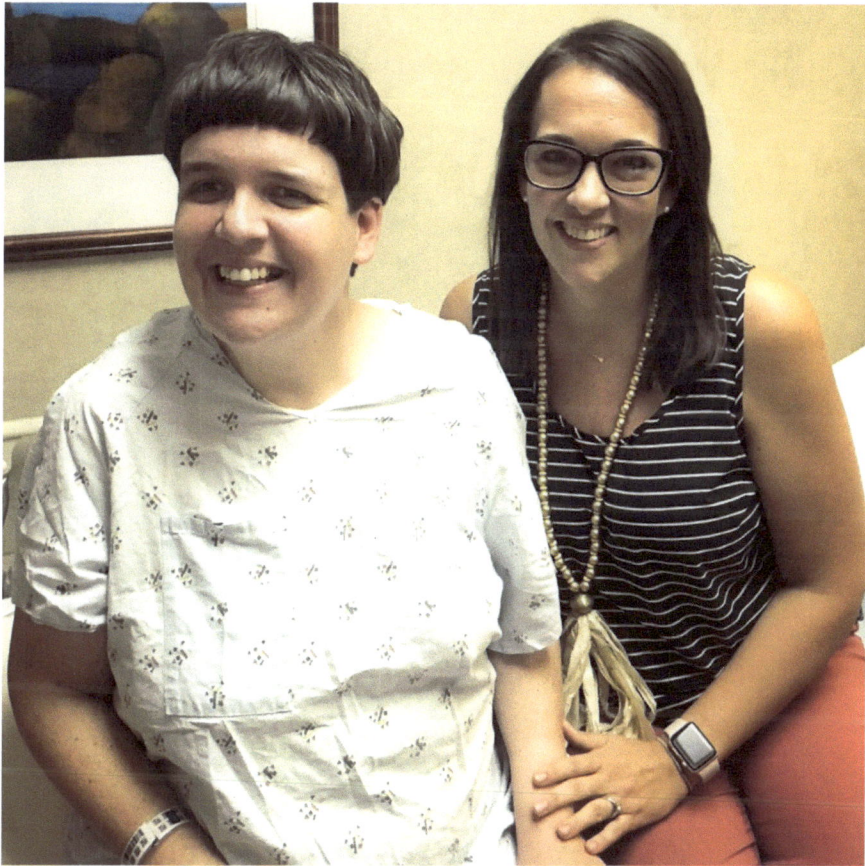

I was taken to the hospital,
because I was so sick.
They put an IV in my arm
with a needle prick.

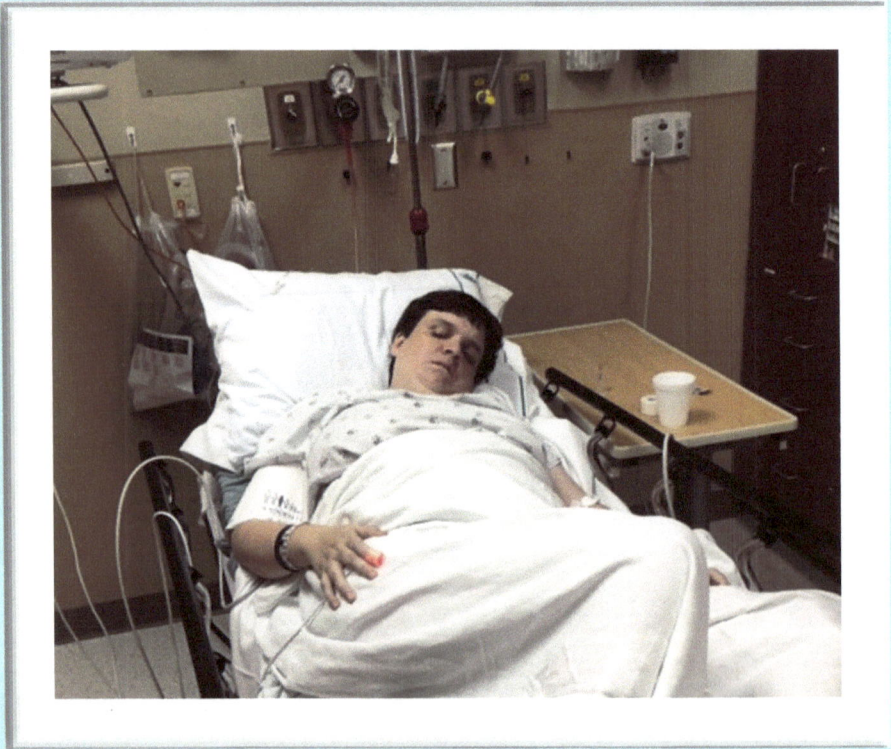

The nurse was very gentle.
It really wasn't bad.
I never even worried—
okay, maybe just a tad.

The IV gave me medicine
that took away the pain.
The gown they let me wear in bed
was comfy and quite plain.

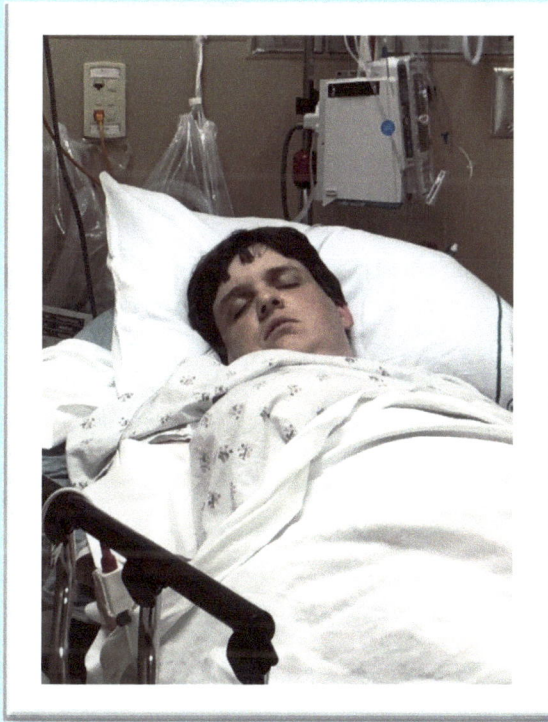

They put a cuff around my arm
that squeezed a little bit.
It made a noise but didn't hurt.
I never minded it.

An ultrasound and CAT scan
were used to take a look
to try and find my problem
from the pictures that they took.

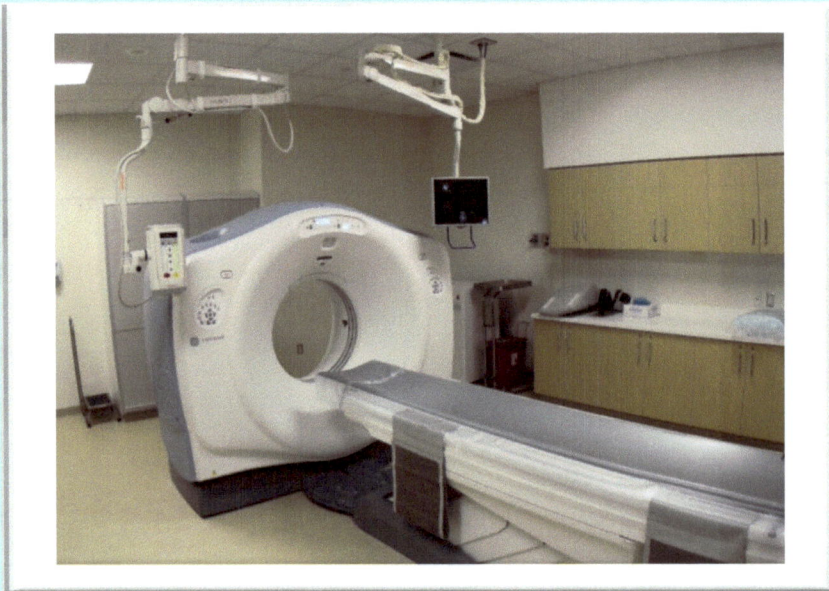

The machines may look quite scary,
but I really didn't care
since they were painless, also,
and my dad was ALWAYS there.

They said I had to spend the night—
more tests they'd have to run.
It might be several days
before they all were finally done.

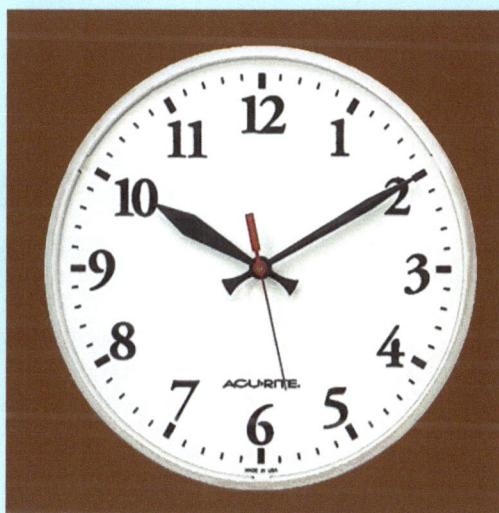

You do a lot of WAITING
when you go through times like these,
but everyone's so thorough
with lots of expertise.

Then they rolled me in my bed
up to another floor.
A BED IN AN ELEVATOR!
I'd not seen that before.

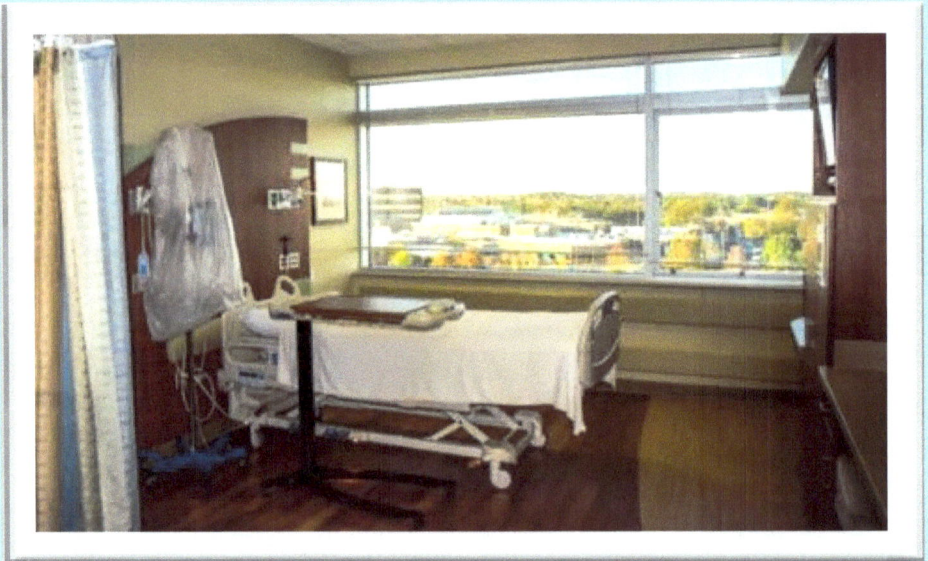

My new room had large windows
with some blinds to cut the glare.
Unlike my room at home,
this one seemed a little bare.

The floor did not have carpet,
but it did look very clean,
and THIS bed had its own remote
to watch the TV screen.

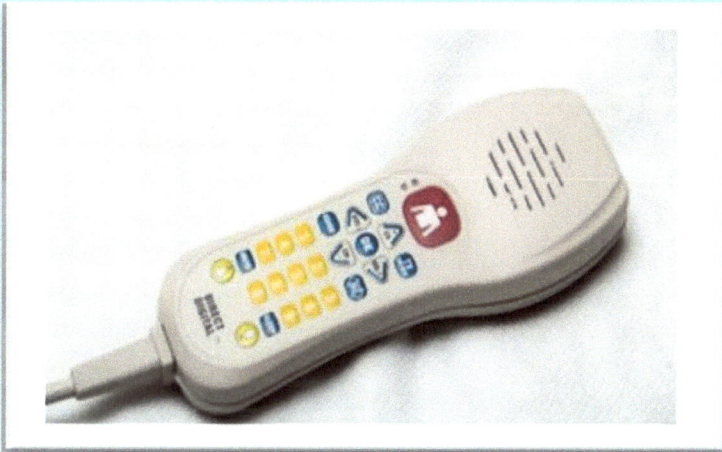

It also had a button
I could press to call a nurse
if anything should happen
or if ever I felt worse.

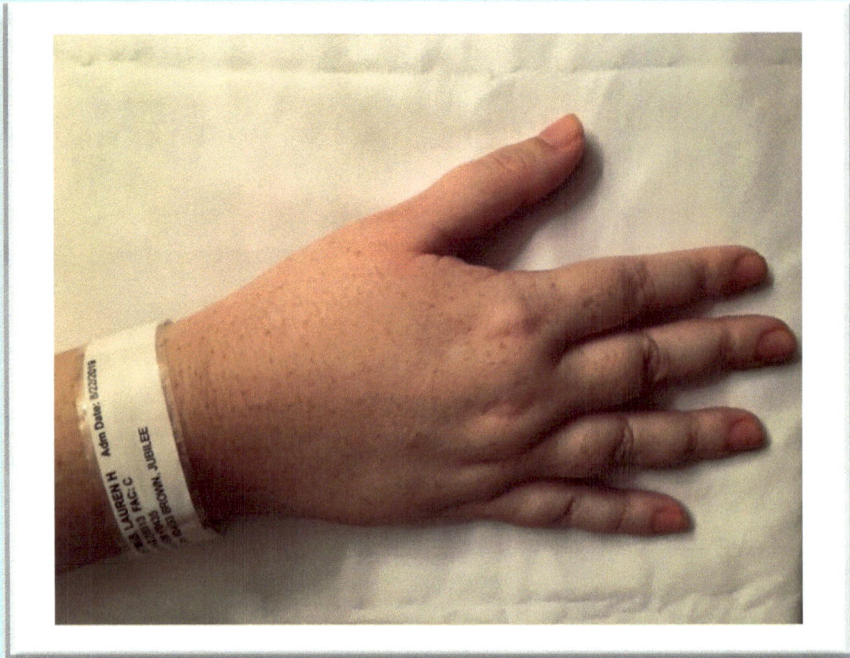

I wore a bracelet on my wrist
that gave them every fact,
like my name and my birthday,
that kept us all on track.

The doctors and the nurses
were all extremely nice.
I wanted to get well,
so I followed their advice.

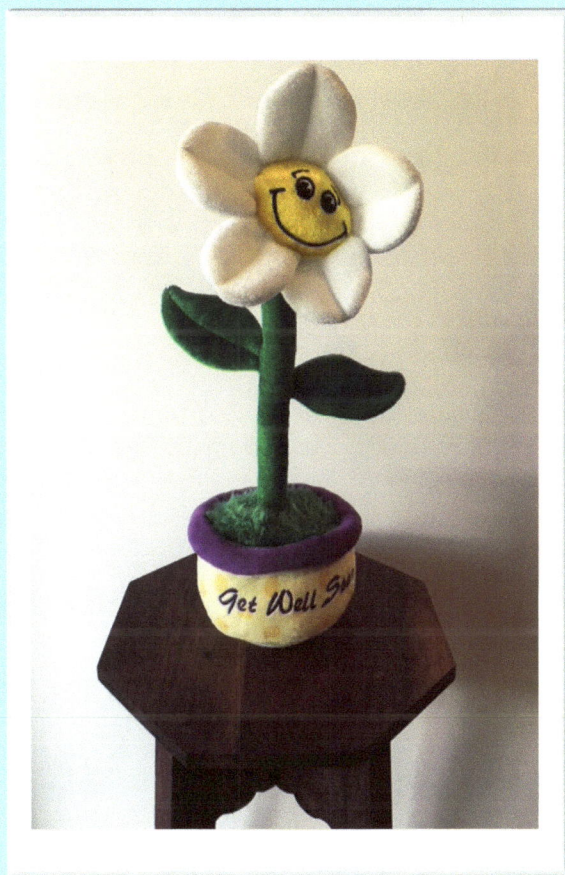

Later, they would tell me
that I had to go downtown,
where I'd see another doctor
whose name was Dr. Brown.

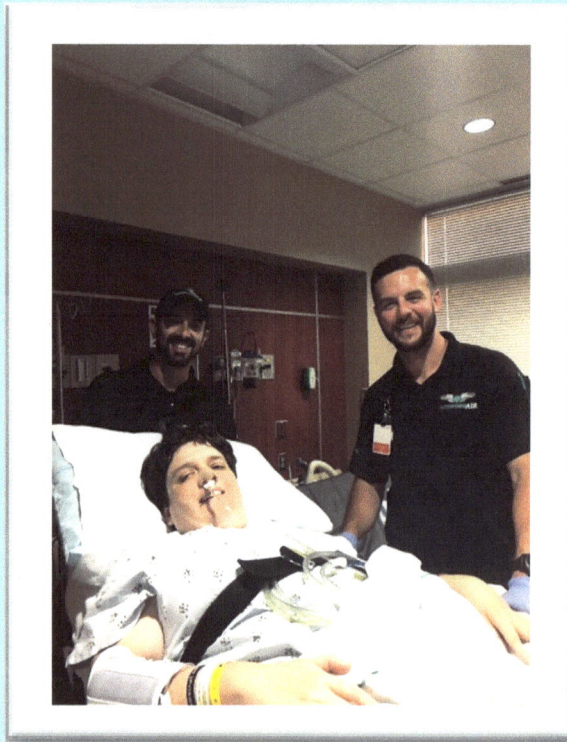

An ambulance would take me
on my trip to this new place.
They strapped me on a stretcher
with a seat belt, just in case.

They gave me extra medicine
in case the ride was rough.
I sort of liked the bouncy trip.
It must have been enough.

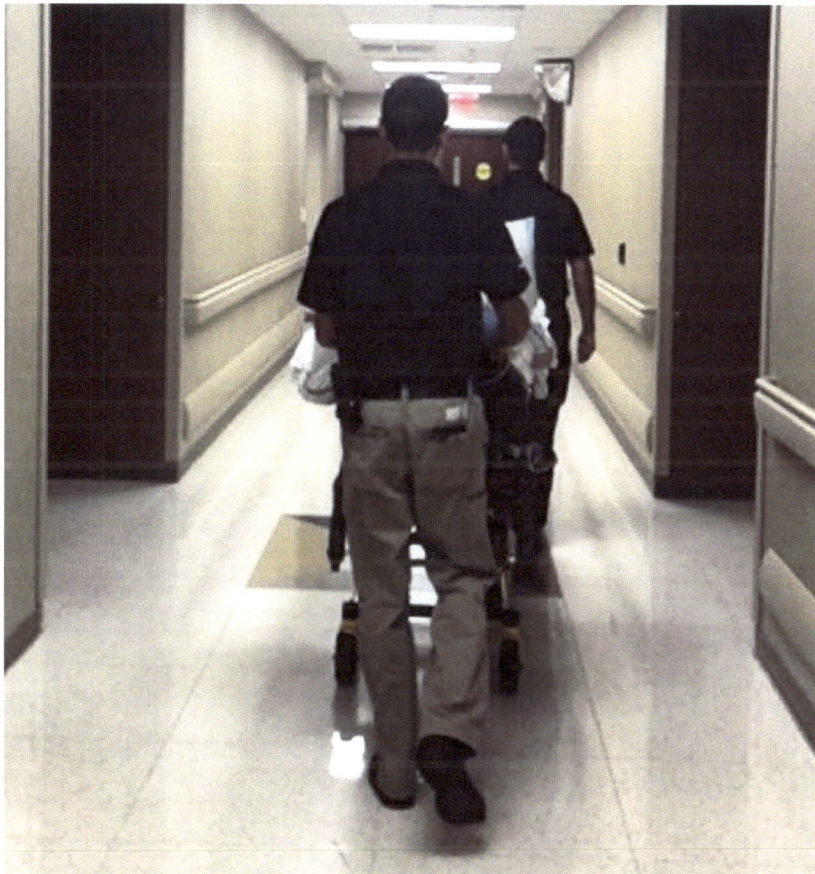

I really liked my doctor.
Jubilee was her first name.
That's a word used in the Bible
when FREEDOM was proclaimed.

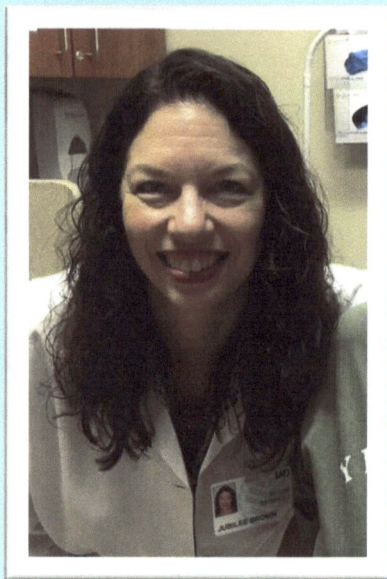

She communicated with me
making sure that all was good,
and even though I cannot talk,
she always understood.

I had a lot of visitors
like my good friend, Ray.
He even came to visit me
on Independence Day.

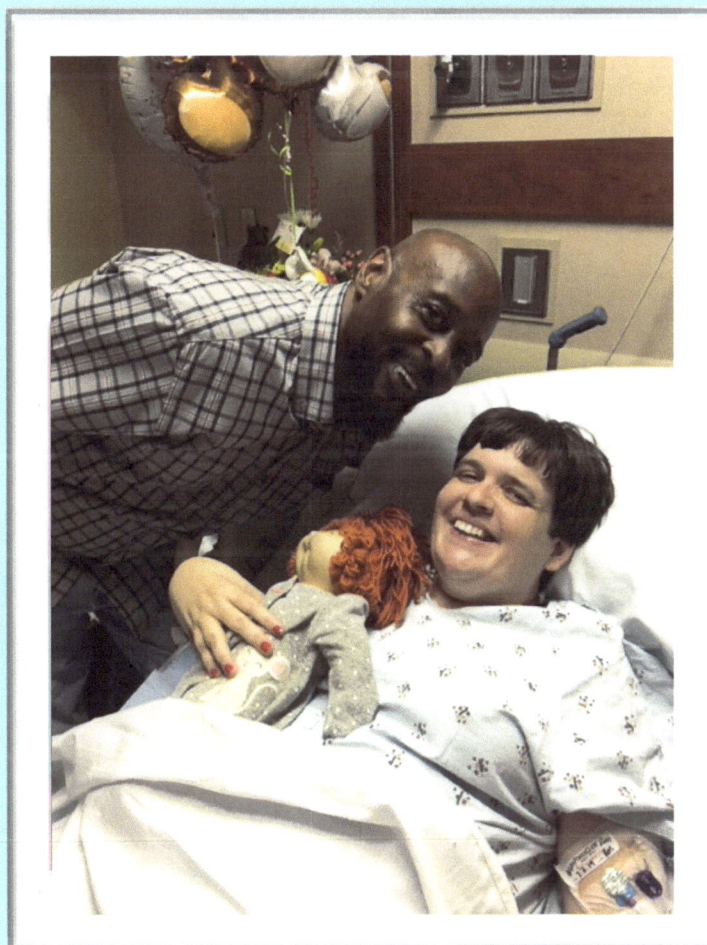

My room became quite crowded
with balloons and gifts galore!
It wasn't very long before
my room was bare NO MORE.

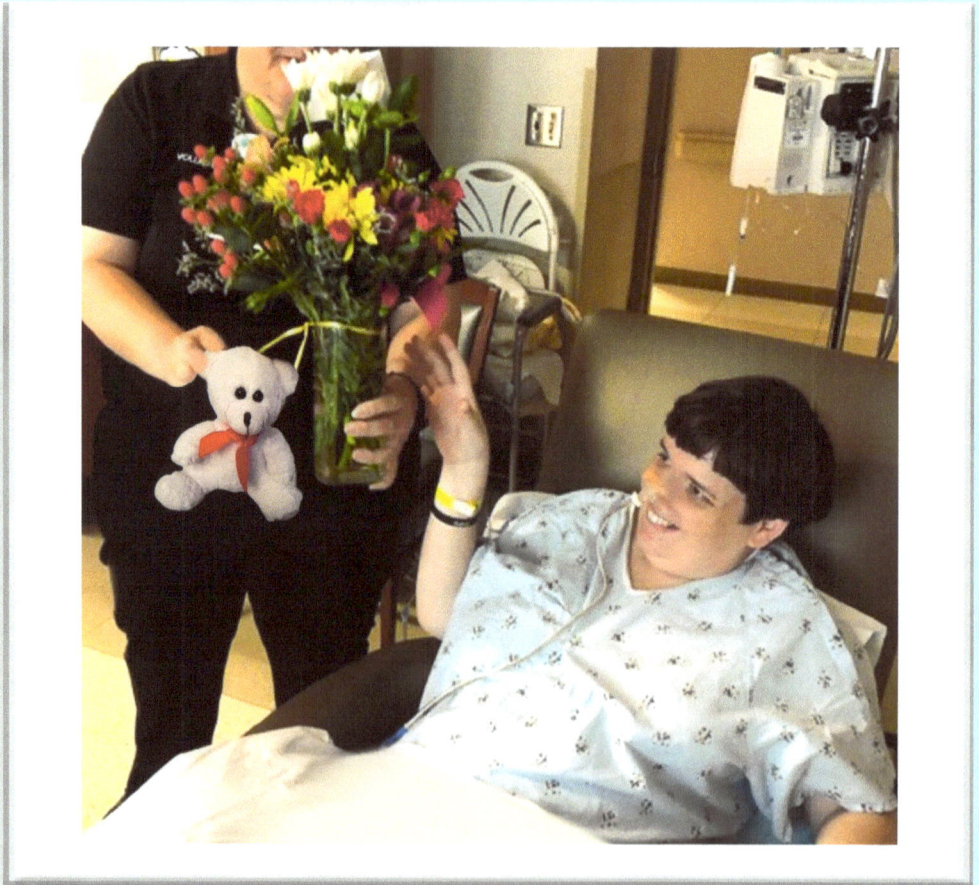

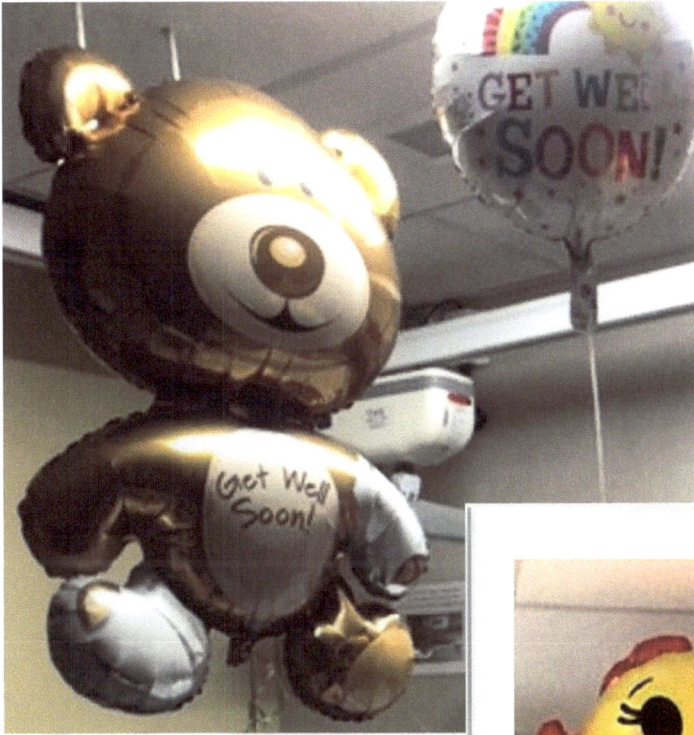
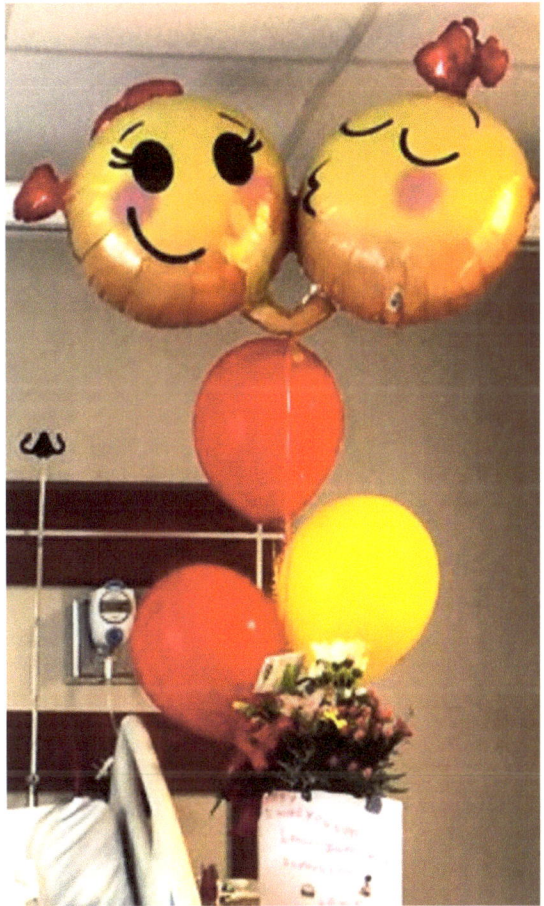

After I went home,
a little later I would see
my doctor in her office
with a need for surgery.

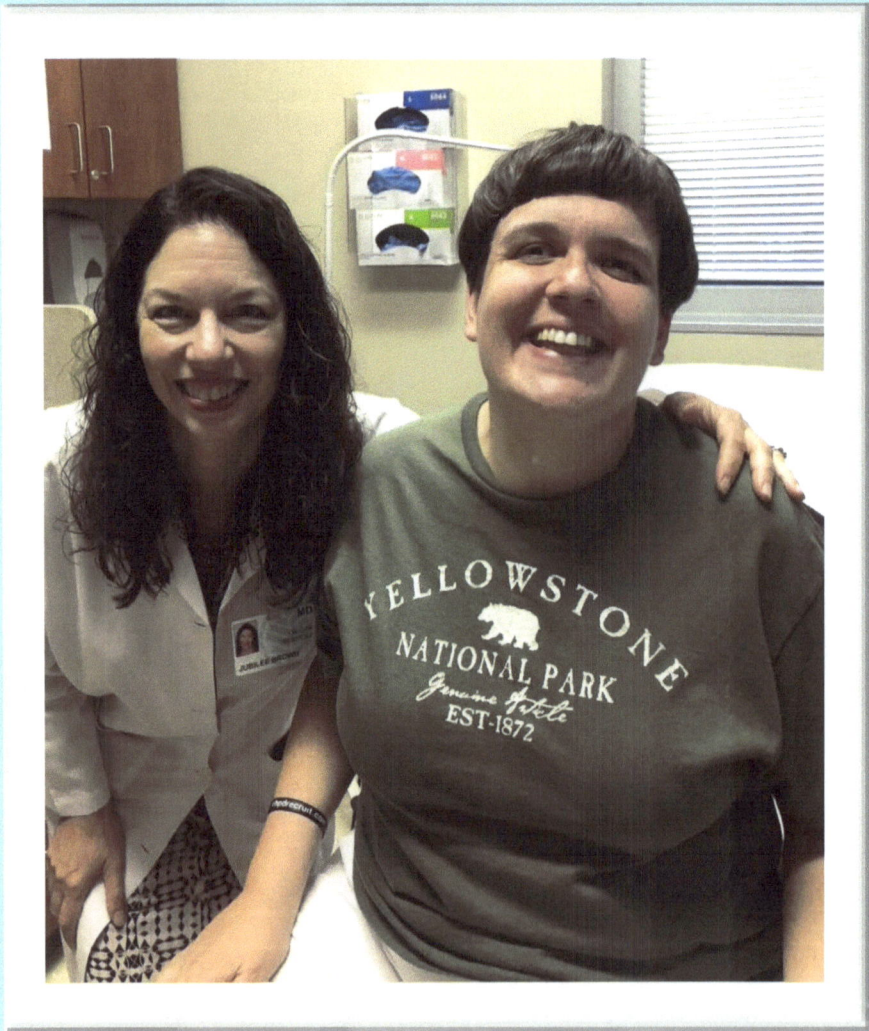

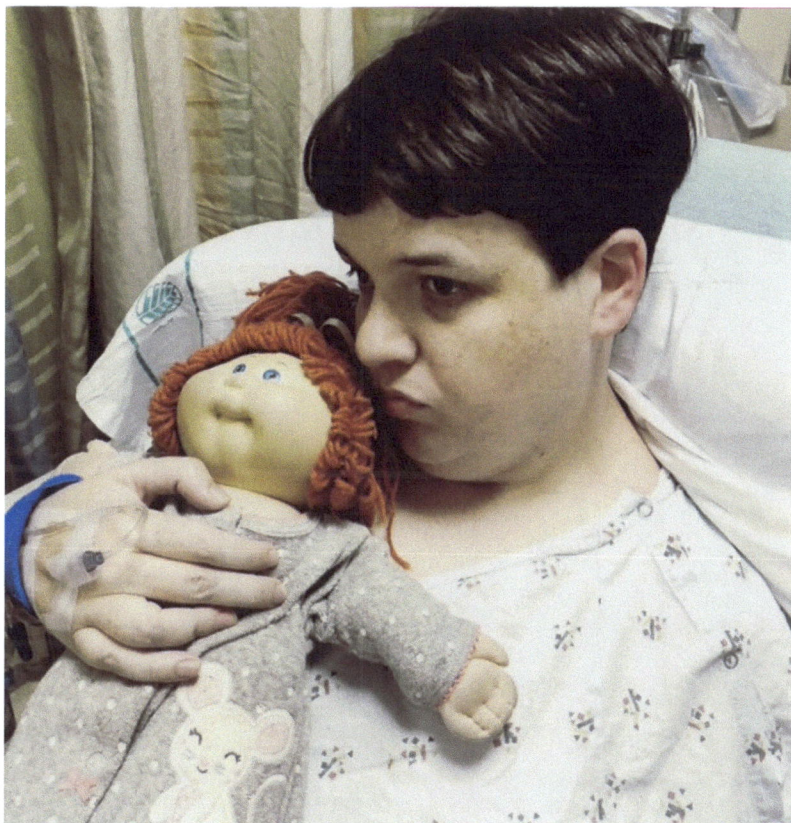

My operation wasn't bad.
I wasn't scared at all.
They told me I could even
bring along my favorite doll.

Waking up took quite a while
when everything was through.
But when I woke and saw my sis,
she knew just what to do.

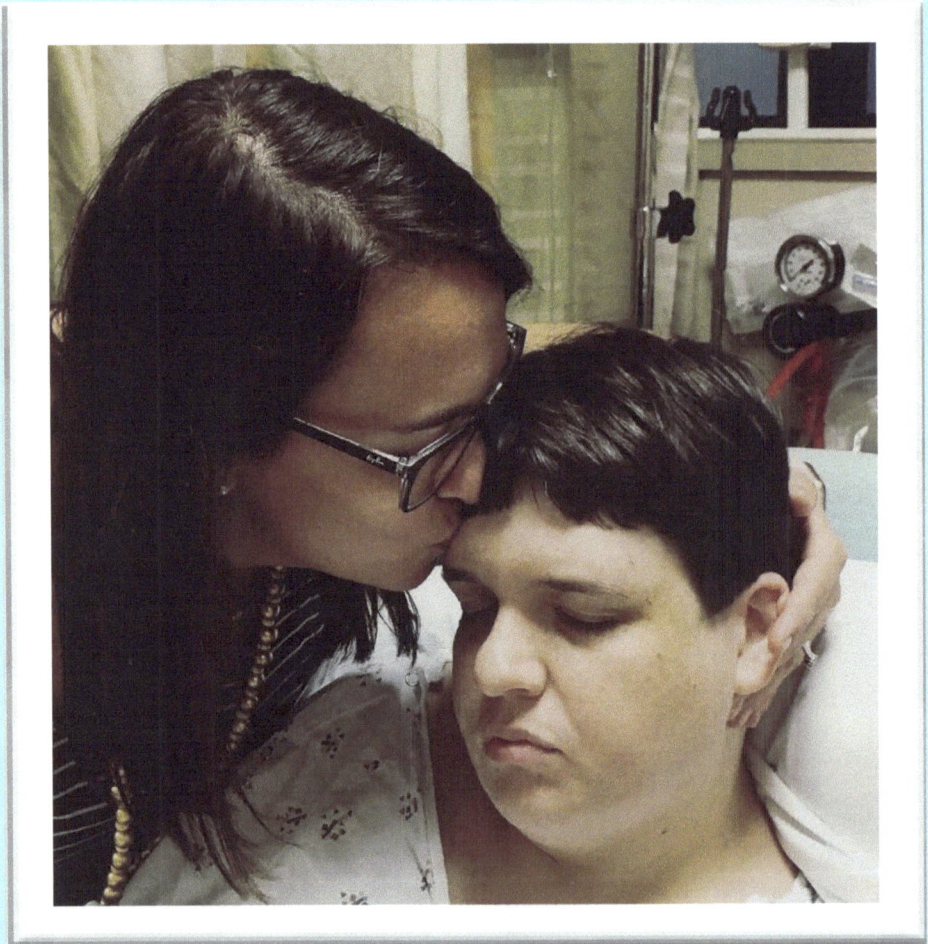

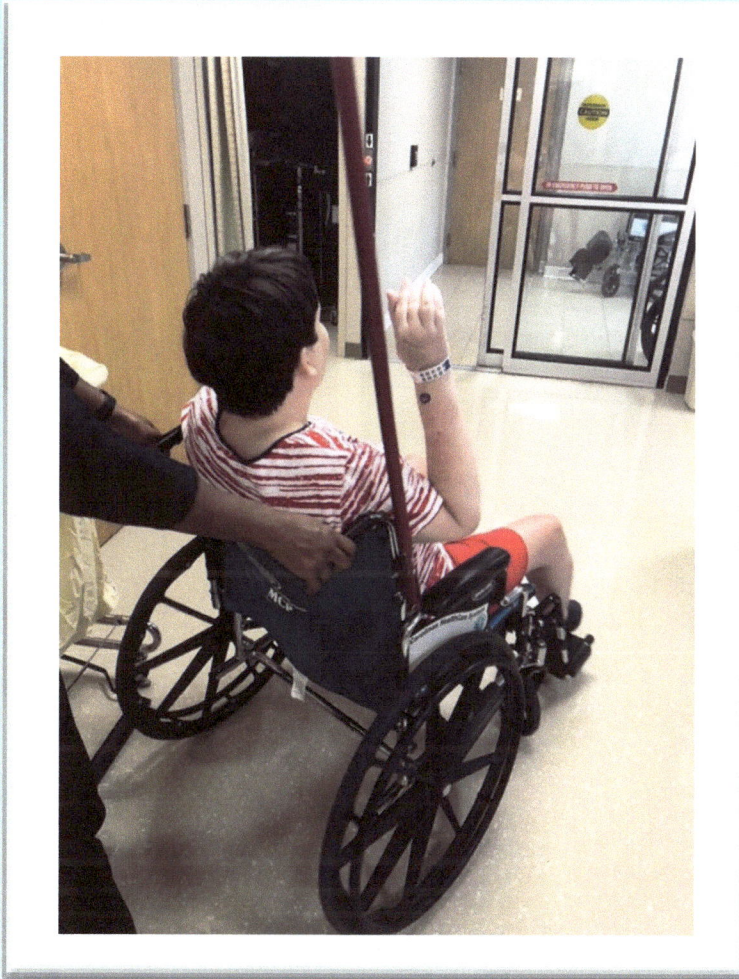

She kissed my face and hugged me
like I was a superstar.
I was helped into a wheelchair
and then rolled to the car.

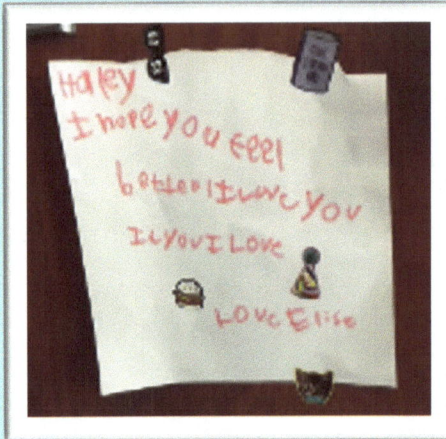

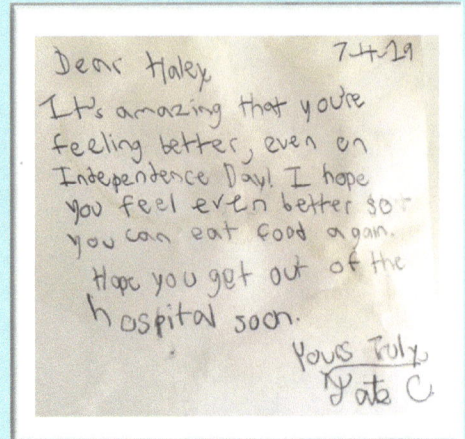

Lots of people prayed for me
and wrote me notes and such.
I knew that I was very loved,
but maybe not **THIS** much!

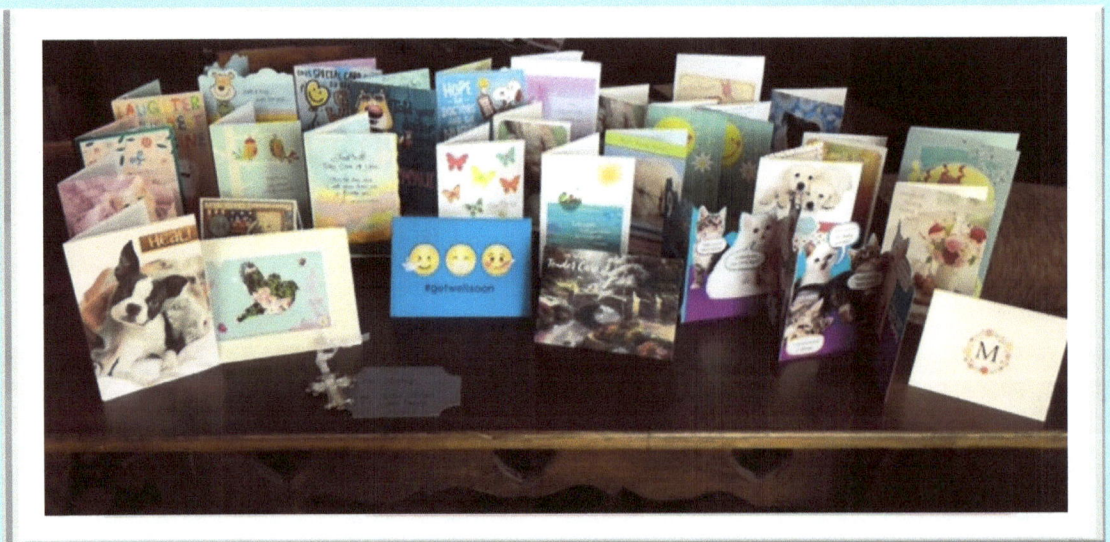

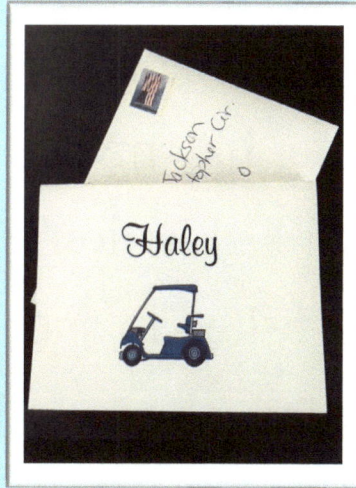

I mailed a lot of thank you cards.

My name was on each one.

My mom would write a note inside,

and I would sign when done.

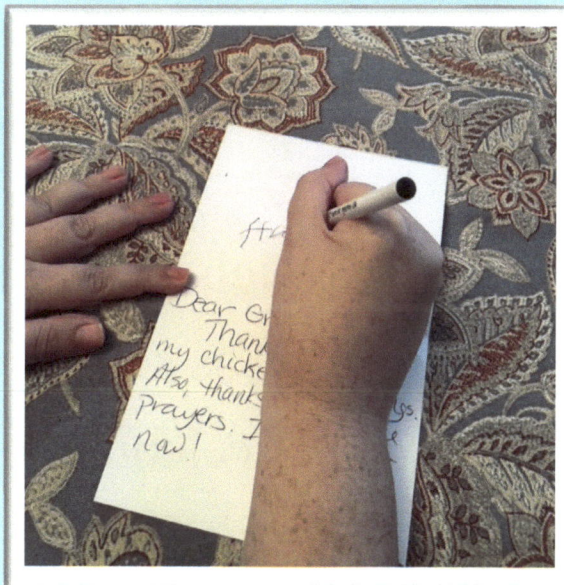

I'm feeling like myself again.

I'm REALLY doing well.

My mom was asked to speak at church.

She had a lot to tell ...

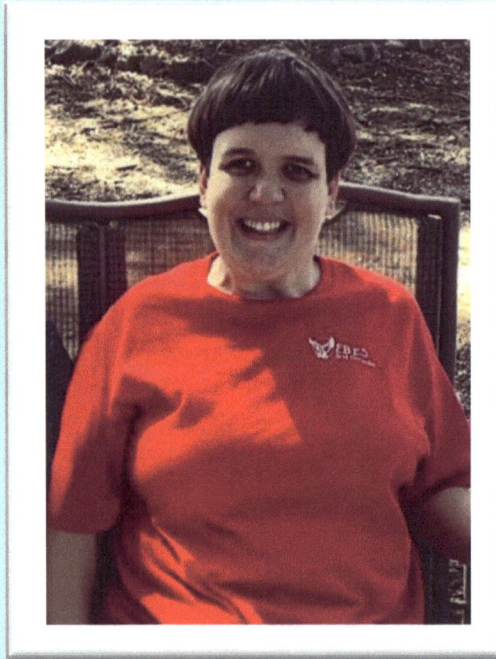

how God completely healed me,

and from pain I was set FREE.

What a time of celebration!

It was my ...

JUBILEE!

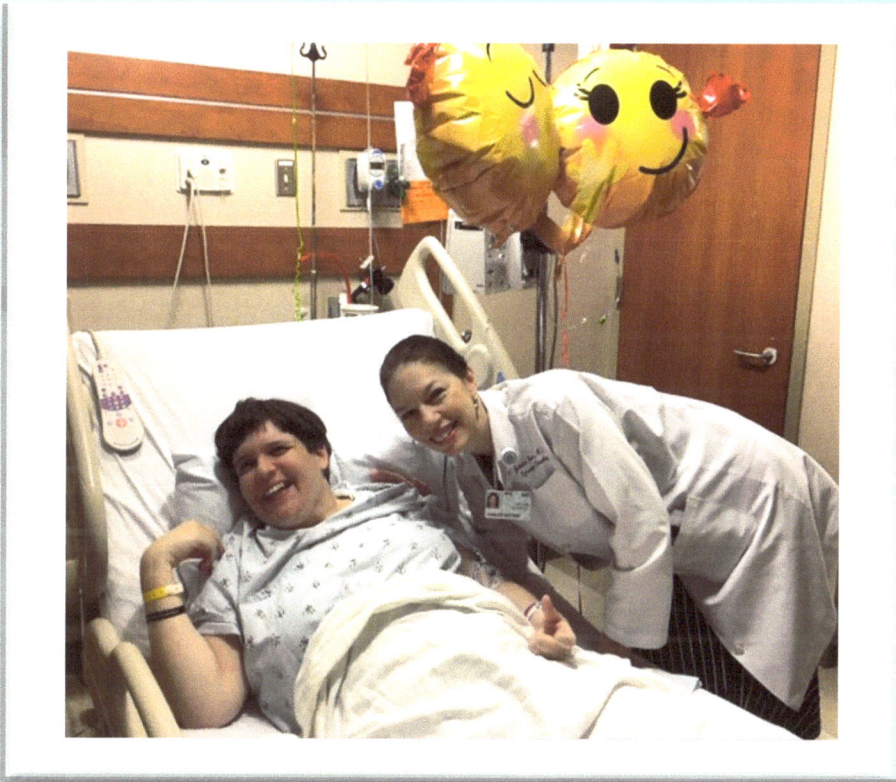

THE END

www.ingramcontent.com/pod-product-compliance
Lightning Source LLC
Chambersburg PA
CBHW060841270326
41933CB00002B/157